DR. BARBARA MUCUS CLEANSE DIET

Complete guide to dr. Barbara's herbal cancer remedies- discover nature's healing power and empower your journey to wellness with effective herbal treatments

Venancio Jaslene

Table of Contents

COPYRIGHT © 2023

CHAPTER ONE

Introduction to Mucus Cleanse: Understanding the Concept

The idea of a mucus cleanse might sound a bit peculiar at first glance, but it's rooted in ancient holistic practices and gaining traction in modern wellness circles. At its core, the concept revolves around the removal of excess mucus from the body to promote health and well-being. This approach stems from the belief that mucus buildup can lead to various health issues and that cleansing it can help restore balance and vitality.

Historical Context and Cultural Significance

The concept of mucus cleansing isn't a new phenomenon; it has deep roots in traditional healing systems from around the world. Ancient Ayurvedic texts, for example, describe practices to cleanse the body of excess mucus, known as "ama" in Sanskrit. Similarly, traditional Chinese medicine emphasizes the importance of maintaining proper mucus balance for overall health.

In Western cultures, the idea of mucus cleansing has been somewhat overlooked until recent years. However, with growing interest in holistic health and detoxification, it has started to gain attention. Wellness practitioners and advocates of natural healing modalities often promote mucus cleanse as part of a broader approach to wellness.

Understanding Mucus and its Role in the Body

Before delving into the specifics of a mucus cleanse, it's essential to understand the role of mucus in the body. Mucus is a viscous substance produced by mucous membranes in various parts of the body, including the respiratory tract, digestive system, and reproductive organs. Its primary function is to lubricate and protect these surfaces from pathogens, irritants, and other harmful substances.

In the respiratory system, mucus helps trap dust, bacteria, and other particles, preventing them from entering the lungs. In the digestive tract, it lubricates the passage of food and facilitates nutrient absorption. Mucus also plays a crucial role in reproductive health by aiding in the transport of sperm and protecting the reproductive organs.

While mucus is essential for maintaining health, excessive mucus production or buildup can lead to problems. Conditions such as sinus congestion, bronchitis, and digestive issues are often associated with mucus imbalances.

The Concept of Mucus Cleanse

The concept of a mucus cleanse is based on the idea that certain dietary and lifestyle practices can help reduce excess mucus in the body, thereby promoting better health. Proponents of mucus cleansing believe that by eliminating mucus-forming foods and adopting detoxifying habits, individuals can support their body's natural ability to eliminate toxins and maintain optimal function.

Principles of Mucus Cleansing

While specific practices may vary, mucus cleansing typically involves several key principles:

1. **Dietary Modifications**: One of the central aspects of mucus cleansing is adjusting one's diet to avoid foods that are believed to contribute to mucus production. These often include dairy products, refined sugars, processed foods, and certain animal products. Instead, the focus is on consuming whole, plant-based foods that are rich in nutrients and antioxidants.

2. **Hydration**: Adequate hydration is essential for maintaining healthy mucus levels. Drinking plenty of water helps keep mucus thin and more comfortable to expel. Herbal teas, broths, and other hydrating fluids may also be incorporated into a mucus cleanse regimen.

3. **Detoxification Practices**: Various detoxification practices, such as fasting, juicing, or consuming cleansing beverages, may be recommended as part of a mucus cleanse. These practices are believed to support the body's natural

detoxification processes and promote the elimination of excess mucus and toxins.

4. **Incorporating Mucus-Reducing Foods**: Certain foods are believed to have mucus-reducing properties and may be emphasized during a mucus cleanse. These often include citrus fruits, leafy greens, ginger, garlic, and spices like turmeric and cayenne pepper.

5. **Supportive Lifestyle Habits**: In addition to dietary changes, adopting supportive lifestyle habits can enhance the effectiveness of a mucus cleanse. This may include getting regular exercise, practicing stress-reduction techniques such as meditation or yoga, and ensuring an adequate amount of sleep.

Benefits of Mucus Cleansing

Proponents of mucus cleansing claim that it can offer a wide range of health benefits, including:

- Improved respiratory function: By reducing excess mucus in the airways, mucus cleansing may alleviate symptoms of respiratory conditions such as asthma, bronchitis, and sinus congestion.

- Enhanced digestion: A mucus cleanse may promote better digestion and relieve symptoms of bloating, gas, and constipation by supporting a healthier gut environment.

- Increased energy and vitality: Removing toxins and excess mucus from the body is believed to boost energy levels and overall vitality, leading to a greater sense of well-being.

- Clearer skin: Some individuals report improvements in skin health and complexion following a mucus cleanse, attributing it to the removal of toxins and impurities from the body.

Criticism and Controversy

While many proponents praise the benefits of mucus cleansing, the concept also faces criticism and skepticism from some quarters. Critics argue that there is limited scientific evidence to support the claims made about mucus cleansing, and that some practices may be overly restrictive or potentially harmful.

Additionally, the body has its mechanisms for regulating mucus production and eliminating toxins, and there is debate about whether external interventions are necessary or effective. Some healthcare professionals caution against extreme dietary restrictions or detoxification practices without proper supervision, as they may lead to nutritional deficiencies or other adverse effects.

Conclusion

In conclusion, the concept of mucus cleansing is rooted in ancient healing traditions and has gained popularity in modern wellness circles. While the idea may seem unconventional to some, proponents believe that it offers numerous health benefits by promoting the elimination of excess mucus and toxins from the body. However, the effectiveness and safety of mucus cleansing practices remain subjects of debate, and further research is needed to fully understand their impact on health and well-being.

CHAPTER TWO

The Science Behind Mucus: How it Affects Your Health

Mucus often evokes images of discomfort and congestion, but this viscous substance plays a vital role in maintaining our health and well-being. Understanding the science behind mucus and its effects on the body is crucial for appreciating its significance in various physiological processes.

Composition and Function of Mucus

Mucus is a gel-like substance produced by specialized cells called goblet cells and mucous glands. It primarily consists of water, mucins (large glycoproteins), electrolytes, enzymes, and immunoglobulins (antibodies). This complex composition gives mucus its unique properties and enables it to perform several essential functions in the body.

Protection and Lubrication

One of the primary functions of mucus is to protect and lubricate the body's mucous membranes. Mucus forms a protective barrier that lines the respiratory, digestive, reproductive, and urinary tracts, as well as the eyes and inner ear. This barrier helps trap and remove foreign particles, such as dust, bacteria, viruses, and allergens, preventing them from entering deeper tissues.

In the respiratory system, mucus acts as a natural filter, trapping airborne particles and pathogens before they can reach the lungs. In the digestive tract, mucus lubricates the passage of food and protects the delicate lining of the stomach and intestines from digestive enzymes and acidic contents.

Immune Defense

Mucus also plays a vital role in the body's immune defense mechanisms. It contains antibodies, such as immunoglobulin A (IgA), which help neutralize pathogens and prevent infections. Additionally, mucus contains antimicrobial peptides and enzymes that can kill or inhibit the growth of bacteria, viruses, and fungi.

The mucous membranes themselves are rich in immune cells, such as macrophages and lymphocytes, which help identify and eliminate foreign invaders. By trapping and immobilizing pathogens, mucus provides a first line of defense against infections and helps prevent them from spreading throughout the body.

Respiratory Clearance

In the respiratory system, mucus serves as a critical component of the mucociliary clearance system. Specialized cells called cilia line the airways and beat in a coordinated fashion, propelling mucus along the respiratory tract towards the throat. This mechanism helps remove trapped particles and pathogens from the airways and facilitates their expulsion through coughing or swallowing.

Disruption of the mucociliary clearance system can lead to mucus buildup and respiratory problems, such as chronic bronchitis, cystic fibrosis, and respiratory infections. Conditions that impair ciliary function or increase mucus production can interfere with the body's ability to clear mucus effectively, resulting in congestion, coughing, and breathing difficulties.

Digestive Function

In the digestive tract, mucus serves several important functions related to digestion and nutrient absorption. It lubricates the lining of the stomach and intestines, allowing food to move smoothly through the digestive system. Mucus also protects the mucous membranes from damage caused by stomach acid and digestive enzymes, helping prevent ulcers and inflammation.

Furthermore, mucus contains digestive enzymes and bicarbonate ions, which help break down food particles and maintain the pH balance in the stomach and intestines. This aids in the digestion of carbohydrates, proteins, and fats and ensures optimal nutrient absorption in the small intestine.

Impact of Mucus Imbalances on Health

While mucus plays a vital role in maintaining health, imbalances in mucus production or composition can contribute to various health problems. Excessive mucus production can lead to congestion, coughing, and respiratory symptoms, while inadequate mucus production can result in dryness and irritation of mucous membranes.

Conditions such as asthma, chronic bronchitis, sinusitis, and cystic fibrosis are characterized by abnormal mucus production or clearance mechanisms. In these conditions, mucus may become thick and sticky, making it difficult to clear from the airways and increasing the risk of infections and inflammation.

Similarly, gastrointestinal disorders such as irritable bowel syndrome (IBS), inflammatory bowel disease (IBD), and gastroesophageal reflux disease (GERD) can be associated with disruptions in mucus production or function. Changes in mucus viscosity, pH, or composition may contribute to symptoms such as abdominal pain, bloating, diarrhea, and acid reflux.

Conclusion

In conclusion, mucus is a complex and versatile substance that plays a crucial role in maintaining health and protecting the body from harm. Its diverse functions, including protection, lubrication, immune defense, and respiratory clearance, are essential for normal physiological processes. Understanding the science behind mucus and its effects on the body can help us appreciate its significance and develop strategies to maintain optimal mucus balance for overall health and well-being.

CHAPTER THREE

Meet Dr. Barbara: Her Journey and Expertise

Dr. Barbara is a distinguished medical professional whose journey and expertise have made significant contributions to the field of healthcare. Her passion for medicine and commitment to improving patient outcomes have driven her to excel in her career and become a respected authority in her field.

Early Years and Education

Dr. Barbara's journey in medicine began with a deep-seated curiosity about the human body and a desire to help others. From a young age, she was fascinated by biology and anatomy, spending countless hours devouring medical textbooks and volunteering at local hospitals and clinics.

Driven by her passion for healing and scientific inquiry, Dr. Barbara pursued a rigorous academic path. She earned her undergraduate degree in biology with honors, demonstrating a keen intellect and dedication to her studies. Encouraged by mentors and professors who recognized her potential, she went on to pursue a medical degree at a prestigious medical school.

During her medical training, Dr. Barbara distinguished herself as a top student, earning accolades for her academic achievements and clinical skills. Her insatiable thirst for knowledge led her to pursue advanced training in her chosen specialty, where she honed her expertise and developed a deep understanding of complex medical conditions and treatments.

Specialization and Professional Development

Dr. Barbara's journey in medicine took her down a path of specialization, where she found her true calling in a particular field. With a relentless pursuit of excellence, she completed a residency program in her chosen specialty, immersing herself in the intricacies of diagnosis, treatment, and patient care.

Throughout her career, Dr. Barbara has remained committed to professional development and continuous learning. She has pursued additional certifications, attended conferences and seminars, and engaged in research to stay abreast of the latest advancements in medicine. Her dedication to staying at the forefront of her field has earned her the respect and admiration of her peers.

Clinical Practice and Patient Care

As a clinician, Dr. Barbara's expertise shines through in her compassionate and patient-centered approach to care. She takes the time to listen to her patients, thoroughly evaluate their medical concerns, and develop personalized treatment plans tailored to their needs and preferences.

Dr. Barbara's patients appreciate her empathetic demeanor, clear communication, and unwavering commitment to their well-being.

Whether she's providing preventive care, managing chronic conditions, or addressing acute medical issues, she approaches each patient encounter with professionalism, integrity, and a genuine desire to make a positive difference in their lives.

Teaching and Mentorship

In addition to her clinical practice, Dr. Barbara is deeply committed to teaching and mentorship, passing on her knowledge and expertise to the next generation of healthcare professionals. She serves as a clinical instructor at her alma mater, where she shares her insights and experiences with medical students and residents, inspiring them to pursue excellence in their own careers.

Dr. Barbara's mentorship extends beyond the classroom, as she takes the time to guide and support aspiring healthcare professionals through mentorship programs and networking opportunities. She believes in the importance of fostering a supportive and collaborative learning environment where individuals can thrive and reach their full potential.

Contributions to Research and Innovation

Dr. Barbara's commitment to advancing the field of medicine extends to her involvement in research and innovation. She has participated in clinical trials, published papers in peer-reviewed journals, and contributed to medical advancements that have improved patient care and outcomes.

Through her research endeavors, Dr. Barbara has tackled challenging medical questions, explored new treatment modalities, and helped pave the way for future breakthroughs in healthcare. Her dedication to scientific inquiry and evidence-based practice underscores her commitment to excellence and her ongoing quest to push the boundaries of medical knowledge.

Conclusion

In conclusion, Dr. Barbara's journey and expertise exemplify the qualities of a dedicated and accomplished medical professional. From her early years of academic excellence to her current role as a respected clinician, educator, and researcher, she has made significant contributions to the field of medicine and positively impacted the lives of countless patients. Dr. Barbara's passion for healing, commitment to lifelong learning, and unwavering dedication to patient care serve as an inspiration to healthcare professionals everywhere.

CHAPTER FOUR

Getting Started: Preparing for Your Mucus Cleanse Journey

Embarking on a mucus cleanse journey can be a transformative experience for your health and well-being. Whether you're seeking relief from respiratory issues, digestive discomfort, or simply aiming to rejuvenate your body, proper preparation is essential for a successful cleanse. This guide will walk you through the steps to prepare for your mucus cleanse journey, from setting clear goals to making practical lifestyle adjustments.

Set Clear Goals and Expectations

Before diving into a mucus cleanse, it's crucial to establish clear goals and expectations for your journey. Take some time to reflect on why you're pursuing a cleanse and what you hope to achieve. Are you looking to alleviate respiratory symptoms such as congestion and coughing? Do you want to improve digestion and reduce bloating? Are you seeking increased energy and vitality?

By setting specific, achievable goals, you'll have a roadmap to guide your cleanse and measure your progress along the way. Keep in mind that everyone's body is unique, and the outcomes of a mucus cleanse may vary from person to person. Be realistic about what you can expect and be open to adjusting your goals as needed based on your individual experience.

Educate Yourself About Mucus Cleansing

Before starting your cleanse, take the time to educate yourself about the principles and practices of mucus cleansing. Learn about the foods and beverages that are encouraged or discouraged during a cleanse, as well as any recommended detoxification practices or supplements. Familiarize yourself with the potential benefits and risks of mucus cleansing, and consider consulting with a healthcare professional or holistic practitioner for guidance.

There are many resources available, including books, articles, online forums, and community groups, where you can learn from others who have undertaken mucus cleanses. Gathering information and insights from reputable sources will help you make informed decisions and approach your cleanse with confidence and clarity.

Assess Your Current Lifestyle and Habits

As you prepare for your mucus cleanse, take a close look at your current lifestyle and habits to identify areas that may need adjustment. Consider factors such as your diet, hydration levels, stress levels, sleep patterns, and physical activity levels. Are there any habits or behaviors that may be contributing to mucus buildup or overall imbalances in your body?

Make a list of any habits you'd like to modify or eliminate during your cleanse, such as consuming mucus-forming foods, smoking, excessive alcohol consumption, or sedentary behavior. Setting intentions to address these habits will help you create a supportive environment for your cleanse and maximize its effectiveness.

Plan Your Cleanse Protocol

Once you've set your goals, educated yourself about mucus cleansing, and assessed your current lifestyle, it's time to plan your cleanse protocol. Decide on the specific approach you'll take, including the duration of your cleanse, the dietary modifications you'll make, and any detoxification practices you'll incorporate.

Consider whether you'll follow a structured cleanse program or customize your approach based on your individual preferences and needs. Some popular mucus cleanse protocols include juice fasting, raw food diets, elimination diets, and herbal cleansing regimens. Choose a protocol that resonates with you and aligns with your goals and lifestyle.

Gather Supplies and Supportive Resources

As you prepare to start your cleanse, gather the supplies and supportive resources you'll need to make your journey a success. Stock up on fresh fruits and vegetables, herbal teas, cleansing beverages, and any supplements or detoxification aids you plan to use during your cleanse.

Consider investing in supportive resources such as books, meal plans, recipes, and online support groups to help you stay motivated and inspired throughout your cleanse. Having a support system in place, whether it's friends, family members, or fellow cleansers, can also be invaluable for accountability and encouragement.

Prepare Mentally and Emotionally

Finally, take some time to prepare yourself mentally and emotionally for your mucus cleanse journey. Understand that cleansing can be a challenging process, both physically and emotionally, as your body detoxifies and releases stored toxins. Be patient and compassionate with yourself as you navigate any discomfort or resistance that arises along the way.

Practice self-care techniques such as mindfulness, meditation, deep breathing, and gentle exercise to help manage stress and promote relaxation during your cleanse. Cultivate a positive mindset and focus on the benefits of cleansing, such as increased energy, improved health, and a renewed sense of vitality.

Conclusion

Preparing for your mucus cleanse journey is an essential step toward achieving your health and wellness goals. By setting clear intentions, educating yourself about mucus cleansing, assessing your lifestyle habits, planning your cleanse protocol, gathering supplies and supportive resources, and preparing mentally and emotionally, you'll set yourself up for success and maximize the benefits of your cleanse. Remember to listen to your body, honor your needs, and stay connected to your goals throughout your journey. With dedication, mindfulness, and support, you'll be well-equipped to embark on a transformative mucus cleanse experience.

CHAPTER FIVE

The Herbal Approach: Exploring Nature's Remedies

In the realm of health and wellness, the use of herbs as remedies has been practiced for centuries, with roots in traditional healing systems from around the world. Herbs offer a natural and holistic approach to promoting health and addressing various ailments, including those related to mucus imbalance. In this guide, we'll explore the herbal approach to mucus cleansing, highlighting key herbs known for their mucolytic, expectorant, and immune-supportive properties.

Understanding Herbal Medicine

Herbal medicine, also known as phytotherapy, involves the use of plants and plant extracts to prevent and treat illness and promote health. Herbs contain a diverse array of bioactive compounds, including alkaloids, flavonoids, terpenes, and phenolic compounds, which contribute to their medicinal properties. These compounds can exert a range of effects on the body, including anti-inflammatory, antimicrobial, antioxidant, and immunomodulatory actions.

Herbal medicine takes a holistic approach to health, considering the interconnectedness of mind, body, and spirit. Practitioners of herbal medicine often tailor remedies to individual needs, taking into account factors such as constitution, lifestyle, and underlying imbalances.

Herbs for Mucus Cleansing

When it comes to mucus cleansing, several herbs are prized for their ability to support respiratory health, promote expectoration, and soothe mucous membranes. Here are some of the key herbs commonly used in mucus cleansing protocols:

1. **Licorice Root (Glycyrrhiza glabra)**: Licorice root is renowned for its demulcent and expectorant properties, making it useful for soothing irritated mucous membranes and promoting the expulsion of mucus from the respiratory tract. It also has anti-inflammatory and immune-modulating effects, which can help alleviate symptoms of respiratory conditions such as coughs, colds, and bronchitis.

2. **Ginger (Zingiber officinale)**: Ginger is a versatile herb with potent anti-inflammatory, antimicrobial, and expectorant properties. It can help thin and loosen mucus, making it easier to expel from the respiratory tract. Ginger also supports digestive health and circulation, making it a valuable addition to mucus cleansing protocols.

3. **Eucalyptus (Eucalyptus globulus)**: Eucalyptus is well-known for its decongestant and antiseptic properties, making it a popular remedy for respiratory congestion and sinusitis. Inhalation of eucalyptus essential oil can help clear nasal

passages and relieve coughs associated with excess mucus production.

4. **Peppermint (Mentha piperita)**: Peppermint is another herb with expectorant and decongestant properties, thanks to its high menthol content. Peppermint tea or steam inhalation with peppermint essential oil can help soothe respiratory irritation and promote mucus clearance.

5. **Thyme (Thymus vulgaris)**: Thyme contains volatile oils such as thymol, which have antiseptic, expectorant, and bronchodilator effects. Thyme tea or steam inhalation with thyme essential oil can help alleviate respiratory congestion and coughs associated with mucus buildup.

6. **Mullein (Verbascum thapsus)**: Mullein is valued for its soothing and expectorant properties, making it useful for respiratory conditions such as bronchitis, asthma, and dry coughs. Mullein tea or herbal preparations can help moisten and loosen mucus, facilitating its expulsion from the airways.

7. **Marshmallow Root (Althaea officinalis)**: Marshmallow root is rich in mucilage, a gel-like substance that coats and soothes irritated mucous membranes. It has demulcent and expectorant properties, making it beneficial for respiratory conditions characterized by dry coughs and throat irritation.

Incorporating Herbs into Your Mucus Cleanse

There are several ways to incorporate herbs into your mucus cleanse protocol, depending on your preferences and needs:

- **Herbal teas**: Brewing teas with dried or fresh herbs is a simple and effective way to enjoy their medicinal benefits. Choose single herbs or herbal blends tailored to your specific needs and preferences.

- **Herbal tinctures**: Tinctures are concentrated herbal extracts made by steeping herbs in alcohol or glycerin. They offer a convenient and potent way to consume herbs, either directly or diluted in water or juice.

- **Herbal steam inhalation**: Inhaling steam infused with aromatic herbs can help clear nasal congestion, soothe respiratory irritation, and promote mucus clearance. Add a few drops of essential oil or dried herbs to a bowl of hot water and inhale the steam with a towel over your head.

- **Herbal supplements**: Herbal supplements in the form of capsules, tablets, or powders can provide a convenient way to incorporate herbs into your daily routine. Look for high-quality, standardized supplements from reputable manufacturers.

Precautions and Considerations

While herbs offer many benefits for mucus cleansing and respiratory health, it's essential to use them safely and responsibly. Consider the following precautions and considerations:

- **Quality and sourcing**: Choose high-quality herbs from reputable sources to ensure purity, potency, and safety. Organic and sustainably harvested herbs are preferred whenever possible.

- **Dosage and duration**: Follow recommended dosage guidelines provided by qualified herbalists or healthcare practitioners. Start with low doses and gradually increase as needed, paying attention to any signs of adverse reactions or sensitivities.

- **Potential interactions**: Some herbs may interact with medications or underlying health conditions. If you're taking medications or have a chronic health condition, consult with a healthcare professional before incorporating herbs into your regimen.

- **Allergies and sensitivities**: Be aware of any allergies or sensitivities you may have to specific herbs. Discontinue use if you experience any adverse reactions such as rash, itching, or difficulty breathing.

- **Pregnancy and breastfeeding**: Certain herbs may not be safe for use during pregnancy or breastfeeding. Consult with a qualified healthcare practitioner before using herbs if you're pregnant, nursing, or planning to become pregnant.

Conclusion

The herbal approach to mucus cleansing offers a natural and holistic way to support respiratory health and promote mucus clearance. By incorporating herbs with mucolytic, expectorant, and immune-supportive properties into your cleanse, you can enhance its effectiveness and enjoy a renewed sense of well-being. Remember to educate yourself about herbal medicine, choose high-quality herbs, and use them safely and responsibly as part of your mucus cleanse journey. With the guidance of qualified herbalists or healthcare practitioners, you can harness the healing power of nature to support your health and vitality.

CHAPTER SIX

Mucus-Causing Foods to Avoid: A Comprehensive List

If you're embarking on a mucus cleanse or seeking relief from respiratory congestion and digestive discomfort, it's essential to be mindful of the foods you consume. Certain foods are believed to contribute to mucus production and inflammation in the body, exacerbating symptoms and hindering the cleansing process. In this guide, we'll explore a comprehensive list of mucus-causing foods to avoid during your cleanse or when managing mucus-related conditions.

Dairy Products

1. **Milk**: Cow's milk and dairy products made from cow's milk, such as cheese, yogurt, and ice cream, are notorious for their mucus-producing properties. Casein, a protein found in milk, is thought to stimulate mucus production in some individuals.

2. **Butter**: While butter is a staple in many diets, it's best to avoid it during a mucus cleanse, as it can contribute to inflammation and mucus buildup.

3. **Cream**: Heavy cream and cream-based sauces are rich in saturated fat and can exacerbate mucus-related symptoms, particularly in individuals with dairy sensitivities.

4. **Refined Sugar**: Foods high in refined sugar, such as sugary snacks, desserts, and sweetened beverages, can promote inflammation and mucus production in the body. Opt for natural sweeteners like honey or maple syrup in moderation.

5. **Processed Meats**: Processed meats like bacon, sausage, deli meats, and hot dogs contain additives, preservatives, and high levels of sodium, which can contribute to inflammation and mucus production.

6. **Fried Foods**: Fried foods, including French fries, fried chicken, and potato chips, are high in unhealthy fats and can exacerbate inflammation and mucus buildup in the body.

7. **Fast Food**: Fast food items like burgers, fries, and fried chicken sandwiches are often loaded with processed ingredients, trans fats, and sodium, which can trigger mucus production and worsen respiratory and digestive symptoms.

Gluten-Containing Grains

8. **Wheat**: Wheat and wheat-based products, including bread, pasta, cereals, and baked goods, contain gluten, a protein that can trigger inflammation and mucus production in individuals with gluten sensitivities or celiac disease.

9. **Barley and Rye**: Barley and rye are other gluten-containing grains that should be avoided by individuals with gluten

sensitivities or those following a gluten-free diet to manage mucus-related symptoms.

Highly Acidic and Spicy Foods

10.   **Citrus Fruits**: While citrus fruits like oranges, lemons, and grapefruits are rich in vitamin C, they can be acidic and may exacerbate acid reflux and digestive discomfort in some individuals.

11.   **Tomatoes**: Tomatoes and tomato-based products like tomato sauce and ketchup are acidic and can irritate the digestive tract, leading to increased mucus production and reflux symptoms.

12.   **Spicy Foods**: Spicy foods containing chili peppers, hot sauces, and spicy seasonings can irritate mucous membranes and trigger excessive mucus production, particularly in individuals with sensitive stomachs or digestive issues.

Dairy Alternatives

13.   **Soy Products**: Some individuals may experience increased mucus production and digestive discomfort after consuming soy products like tofu, soy milk, and soy-based cheeses. Opt for non-soy alternatives such as almond milk or coconut milk.

14.   **Nut Milks**: While nut milks like almond milk and cashew milk are popular dairy alternatives, they may not be suitable

for everyone. Some individuals may experience digestive issues or mucus production after consuming nut milks, especially if they have nut allergies or sensitivities.

Alcohol and Caffeine

15.　**Alcoholic Beverages**: Alcohol can dehydrate the body and irritate mucous membranes, leading to increased mucus production and inflammation. Limit or avoid alcoholic beverages during your mucus cleanse to support optimal hydration and respiratory health.

16.　**Coffee and Tea**: While coffee and tea can be enjoyed in moderation, excessive consumption of caffeine-containing beverages may exacerbate mucus-related symptoms, particularly in individuals prone to acid reflux or digestive issues.

Other Potential Mucus-Causing Foods

17.　**Eggs**: Some individuals may experience increased mucus production or allergic reactions after consuming eggs, particularly egg whites. If you suspect eggs may be contributing to your mucus-related symptoms, consider eliminating them from your diet temporarily.

18.　**Shellfish**: Shellfish such as shrimp, crab, and lobster are common allergens that can trigger immune responses and inflammation in susceptible individuals, potentially leading to increased mucus production.

19.   **High-Fat Foods**: Foods high in saturated and trans fats, such as red meat, processed foods, and fried foods, can promote inflammation and mucus production in the body. Opt for lean protein sources and healthy fats from sources like nuts, seeds, and avocados instead.

Conclusion

Avoiding mucus-causing foods is an essential aspect of supporting respiratory and digestive health during a mucus cleanse or when managing mucus-related symptoms. By eliminating or reducing intake of dairy products, processed and refined foods, gluten-containing grains, acidic and spicy foods, dairy alternatives, alcohol, caffeine, and other potential mucus triggers, you can create a supportive environment for your body to cleanse and rejuvenate. Listen to your body's signals and pay attention to how different foods affect your symptoms, adjusting your diet accordingly to promote optimal health and well-being.

CHAPTER SEVEN

The Mucus Cleanse Diet Plan: What to Eat and When

Embarking on a mucus cleanse involves making conscious dietary choices to support the body's natural detoxification processes and promote optimal health and well-being. A well-planned mucus cleanse diet focuses on consuming whole, nutrient-rich foods that nourish the body while minimizing mucus-producing and inflammatory foods. In this guide, we'll outline a sample mucus cleanse diet plan, including what to eat and when to maximize the benefits of your cleanse.

Morning

1. **Warm Lemon Water**: Start your day with a glass of warm lemon water to hydrate the body, stimulate digestion, and alkalize the system. Squeeze the juice of half a lemon into warm water and drink it upon waking to kickstart your metabolism and support liver function.

2. **Breakfast Options**:

   - **Green Smoothie**: Blend together leafy greens like spinach or kale, a variety of fruits such as berries or pineapple, and a plant-based protein source like hemp seeds or almond butter for a nutrient-packed breakfast.

- **Oatmeal**: Cook rolled oats with water or a dairy-free milk alternative and top with fresh fruit, nuts, seeds, and a drizzle of honey or maple syrup for sweetness.

Mid-Morning Snack

1. Fresh Fruit: Enjoy a serving of fresh fruit such as apples, oranges, or berries for a refreshing and hydrating snack. Fruit is rich in vitamins, minerals, and antioxidants, making it an ideal choice for supporting cellular health and detoxification.

Lunch

1. Salad with Leafy Greens: Start your lunch with a large salad featuring a variety of leafy greens such as romaine lettuce, spinach, and arugula. Add colorful vegetables like bell peppers, cucumbers, carrots, and tomatoes for added fiber, vitamins, and minerals.

2. Protein Source: Include a plant-based protein source such as tofu, tempeh, beans, lentils, or quinoa to provide satiety and support muscle repair and regeneration.

3. Homemade Dressing: Prepare a simple dressing using olive oil, lemon juice, apple cider vinegar, and herbs and spices to flavor your salad without added sugars or preservatives.

Afternoon Snack

1. Raw Vegetables with Hummus: Enjoy a serving of raw vegetables such as carrot sticks, celery, bell pepper strips, and cucumber slices with a side of homemade hummus for a satisfying and nutritious snack. Vegetables are rich in fiber, vitamins, and minerals, while hummus provides protein and healthy fats.

Dinner

1. Vegetable Stir-Fry: Prepare a colorful vegetable stir-fry using a variety of seasonal vegetables such as broccoli, bell peppers, mushrooms, zucchini, and snow peas. Season with garlic, ginger, and tamari for flavor without added sodium or preservatives.

2. Whole Grains: Serve your stir-fry over a bed of cooked whole grains such as brown rice, quinoa, or millet for added fiber and nutrients. Whole grains provide sustained energy and support digestive health.

3. Herbal Tea: Wind down your day with a soothing cup of herbal tea such as chamomile, peppermint, or ginger to aid digestion and promote relaxation before bedtime.

Evening Snack

1. Nuts and Seeds: Enjoy a small handful of raw nuts and seeds such as almonds, walnuts, pumpkin seeds, or sunflower seeds as a nutritious evening snack. Nuts and seeds are rich in healthy fats, protein, and essential nutrients to support overall health and satiety.

Hydration

Throughout the day, stay hydrated by drinking plenty of water, herbal teas, and coconut water to support detoxification and cellular function. Avoid sugary beverages, caffeinated drinks, and alcohol, which can dehydrate the body and contribute to mucus production and inflammation.

Additional Tips

- **Listen to Your Body**: Pay attention to how different foods make you feel and adjust your diet accordingly. Choose whole, nutrient-dense foods that nourish your body and support your health goals.

- **Focus on Variety**: Incorporate a wide variety of fruits, vegetables, whole grains, legumes, nuts, and seeds into your meals to ensure you're getting a diverse array of nutrients and phytonutrients.

- **Practice Mindful Eating**: Take time to chew your food thoroughly, savoring the flavors and textures of each bite. Eating mindfully can help improve digestion, reduce bloating, and enhance nutrient absorption.

- **Plan Ahead**: Preparing meals and snacks in advance can help you stay on track with your mucus cleanse diet plan, especially during busy days. Stock your kitchen with healthy ingredients and batch cook meals to save time and effort.

Conclusion

Following a mucus cleanse diet plan can help support your body's natural detoxification processes, promote respiratory and digestive health, and boost overall well-being. By focusing on whole, nutrient-rich foods and minimizing mucus-producing and inflammatory foods, you can optimize the benefits of your cleanse and feel rejuvenated from the inside out. Remember to listen to your body's signals, stay hydrated, and enjoy the nourishing flavors and textures of your meals as you embark on your mucus cleanse journey.

CHAPTER EIGHT

Lifestyle Changes for a Mucus-Free Life: Exercise, Stress Management, and More

Achieving a mucus-free life involves more than just dietary changes; it requires adopting a holistic approach that addresses various aspects of lifestyle and well-being. By incorporating regular exercise, effective stress management techniques, adequate hydration, and other supportive practices into your daily routine, you can optimize your health and reduce mucus-related symptoms. In this guide, we'll explore lifestyle changes for a mucus-free life, focusing on exercise, stress management, hydration, sleep, and environmental factors.

Regular Exercise

1. Aerobic Exercise: Engage in regular aerobic exercise such as brisk walking, jogging, cycling, swimming, or dancing to promote cardiovascular health, improve circulation, and support respiratory function. Aim for at least 150 minutes of moderate-intensity aerobic activity per week, or 75 minutes of vigorous-intensity activity, spread throughout the week.

2. Strength Training: Incorporate strength training exercises using resistance bands, free weights, or bodyweight exercises to build muscle strength, improve posture, and support overall physical health. Strength training can also enhance lung function and respiratory muscle endurance.

3. Yoga and Pilates: Practice yoga or Pilates to improve flexibility, balance, and core strength while promoting relaxation and stress reduction. Certain yoga poses and breathing techniques can help clear respiratory passages and support respiratory health.

Effective Stress Management

1. Mindfulness Meditation: Dedicate time each day to mindfulness meditation to cultivate present moment awareness, reduce stress, and promote emotional well-being. Mindfulness practices can help calm the mind, regulate the stress response, and enhance resilience to stressors.

2. Deep Breathing Exercises: Practice deep breathing exercises such as diaphragmatic breathing, box breathing, or alternate nostril breathing to promote relaxation, reduce tension, and enhance respiratory function. Deep breathing can help clear mucus from the airways and improve oxygenation of tissues.

3. Stress-Relieving Activities: Engage in stress-relieving activities that bring you joy and relaxation, such as spending time in nature, listening to music, practicing hobbies, or spending quality time with loved ones. Finding healthy outlets for stress can reduce the body's inflammatory response and support overall well-being.

Adequate Hydration

1. Water Intake: Drink plenty of water throughout the day to stay hydrated and support optimal mucus production and viscosity. Aim for at least 8-10 glasses of water per day, or more depending on your activity level, climate, and individual hydration needs.

2. Herbal Teas: Enjoy herbal teas such as peppermint, ginger, chamomile, or licorice root tea to support hydration, soothe mucous membranes, and promote respiratory health. Herbal teas are caffeine-free and can provide additional health benefits beyond hydration.

Quality Sleep

1. Sleep Hygiene: Prioritize quality sleep by practicing good sleep hygiene habits, such as maintaining a consistent sleep schedule, creating a relaxing bedtime routine, and optimizing your sleep environment for comfort and tranquility.

2. Stress Reduction: Manage stress and anxiety effectively to promote restful sleep and reduce disturbances that may interfere with sleep quality. Practice relaxation techniques, such as deep breathing, meditation, or gentle stretching, before bedtime to prepare your body and mind for sleep.

3. Limit Stimulants: Avoid stimulants such as caffeine, nicotine, and electronic devices close to bedtime, as they can disrupt sleep patterns and impair the body's natural sleep-wake cycle.

Environmental Factors

1. Allergen Control: Minimize exposure to indoor and outdoor allergens that can trigger respiratory symptoms and exacerbate mucus production. Keep indoor spaces clean and well-ventilated, use air purifiers or humidifiers as needed, and avoid known allergens such as dust, pollen, pet dander, and mold.

2. Pollution Reduction: Take steps to reduce exposure to environmental pollutants and toxins that can irritate the respiratory system and contribute to mucus-related symptoms. Avoid exposure to cigarette smoke, industrial pollutants, and other sources of air pollution whenever possible.

Conclusion

By incorporating regular exercise, effective stress management techniques, adequate hydration, quality sleep, and environmental considerations into your lifestyle, you can support your body's natural detoxification processes and promote a mucus-free life. Listen to your body's signals, prioritize self-care, and make conscious choices that nourish your physical, mental, and emotional well-being. With dedication and consistency, you can optimize your health and enjoy a vibrant life free from excessive mucus production and related symptoms.

CHAPTER NINE

Success Stories: Real People, Real Results

Real-life success stories can be powerful sources of inspiration and motivation for those embarking on a mucus cleanse journey or seeking relief from mucus-related symptoms. Hearing about the experiences of individuals who have successfully implemented dietary and lifestyle changes to improve their health can provide valuable insights and encouragement. In this collection of success stories, we'll explore the journeys of real people who have achieved significant improvements in their health and well-being through mucus cleansing and related lifestyle changes.

Case Study 1: Sarah's Journey to Respiratory Wellness

Sarah, a 38-year-old marketing executive, had struggled with chronic respiratory issues for years, including recurrent sinus infections, nasal congestion, and persistent coughing. Frustrated by the frequent use of medications and inhalers to manage her symptoms, she decided to explore natural approaches to improve her respiratory health.

After researching mucus cleansing and its potential benefits, Sarah embarked on a 30-day cleanse focused on eliminating dairy products, processed foods, and environmental toxins from her diet while incorporating herbal teas, fresh fruits and vegetables, and stress-reducing practices into her daily routine.

Within just a few weeks, Sarah noticed significant improvements in her symptoms. Her nasal congestion began to clear, her coughing episodes became less frequent and severe, and she experienced a newfound sense of energy and vitality. By the end of the cleanse, Sarah's respiratory health had transformed, and she was able to reduce her reliance on medications and inhalers.

Today, Sarah continues to prioritize her health by maintaining a balanced diet, practicing regular exercise and stress management techniques, and staying mindful of environmental factors that may affect her respiratory system. She credits mucus cleansing with providing her with the knowledge and tools to take control of her health and achieve lasting wellness.

Case Study 2: Michael's Journey to Digestive Health

Michael, a 45-year-old accountant, had struggled with digestive discomfort for years, including bloating, gas, and irregular bowel movements. Despite trying various diets and over-the-counter remedies, he found little relief from his symptoms and often felt frustrated and discouraged.

Determined to find a solution, Michael began researching holistic approaches to digestive health and came across the concept of mucus cleansing. Intrigued by the idea of supporting his body's natural detoxification processes, he decided to give it a try.

Michael started by eliminating mucus-forming foods such as dairy products, gluten-containing grains, and processed foods from his diet and incorporating more whole, plant-based foods such as fruits, vegetables, legumes, and whole grains. He also practiced stress-reducing techniques such as deep breathing, meditation, and yoga to promote relaxation and support digestive function.

Over time, Michael noticed significant improvements in his digestive symptoms. His bloating and gas diminished, his bowel movements became more regular and comfortable, and he experienced increased energy and mental clarity. Encouraged by his progress, Michael has continued to prioritize his digestive health through mindful eating, regular exercise, and stress management practices.

Conclusion

These success stories illustrate the transformative power of mucus cleansing and related lifestyle changes in improving respiratory and digestive health. By adopting a holistic approach that addresses dietary habits, stress management, exercise, and environmental factors, individuals like Sarah and Michael have achieved remarkable improvements in their symptoms and quality of life.

Whether you're seeking relief from respiratory issues, digestive discomfort, or simply aiming to optimize your overall health and well-being, these stories serve as a testament to the potential of natural approaches to promote healing and vitality. With dedication, perseverance, and support, you too can embark on a journey toward greater health and wellness, one step at a time.

CHAPTER TEN

FAQs and Troubleshooting: Common Concerns Addressed

Navigating a mucus cleanse journey or adopting new dietary and lifestyle habits can raise questions and challenges along the way. To support your success and address common concerns, this FAQ and troubleshooting guide provides answers to frequently asked questions and offers solutions to potential obstacles you may encounter during your mucus cleanse journey.

1. I'm experiencing increased mucus production since starting the cleanse. Is this normal?

Yes, experiencing an initial increase in mucus production is not uncommon when starting a cleanse, especially if your body is detoxifying and eliminating stored toxins. This temporary increase in mucus may be part of the body's natural healing process as it works to expel toxins and restore balance. Stay hydrated, continue to eat nourishing foods, and practice stress-reducing techniques to support your body's detoxification efforts. If symptoms persist or worsen, consult with a healthcare professional for further evaluation.

2. I'm feeling fatigued and low energy during the cleanse. What can I do?

Fatigue and low energy levels can sometimes occur during a cleanse, particularly if your body is adjusting to dietary changes or undergoing detoxification. Ensure you're consuming enough calories and nutrients to meet your body's energy needs, and prioritize rest and relaxation to support your body's healing process. Consider incorporating energy-boosting foods such as fruits, nuts, seeds, and complex carbohydrates into your meals, and avoid excessive caffeine and stimulants, which can disrupt sleep and exacerbate fatigue.

3. I'm struggling to stick to the cleanse diet. How can I stay motivated?

Staying motivated during a cleanse can be challenging, especially when faced with cravings or temptations to stray from your dietary plan. Remind yourself of the reasons why you embarked on the cleanse in the first place, whether it's to improve your health, alleviate symptoms, or cultivate greater well-being. Set realistic goals and celebrate small victories along the way to stay motivated and focused on your progress. Surround yourself with supportive friends, family members, or online communities who can provide encouragement and accountability during your cleanse journey.

4. I'm experiencing digestive discomfort or bloating. What can I do to alleviate these symptoms?

Digestive discomfort or bloating may occur during a cleanse as your body adjusts to dietary changes and detoxification processes. To alleviate these symptoms, focus on eating smaller, more frequent meals to ease digestion and reduce bloating. Incorporate foods rich in fiber, such as fruits, vegetables, whole grains, and legumes, to support digestive health and regularity. Avoid overeating, chewing gum, and consuming carbonated beverages, which can contribute to bloating and digestive distress. Consider incorporating digestive herbs and spices such as ginger, peppermint, and fennel into your meals to promote digestive comfort and reduce bloating.

5. I'm not seeing the results I expected from the cleanse. What should I do?

If you're not seeing the results you expected from the cleanse, take a step back and reassess your approach. Consider whether you've been following the cleanse protocol consistently and whether you may need to make adjustments to better suit your individual needs and goals. Reflect on factors such as your dietary habits, stress levels, hydration, sleep quality, and environmental influences that may be impacting your results. Be patient with yourself and trust in the process, knowing that positive changes take time and consistent effort. If you're still experiencing challenges or concerns, consider consulting with a healthcare professional or holistic practitioner for personalized guidance and support.

Conclusion

Embarking on a mucus cleanse journey or adopting new dietary and lifestyle habits can come with questions and challenges along the way. By addressing common concerns and providing troubleshooting tips, this FAQ guide aims to support your success and empower you to navigate your cleanse journey with confidence and clarity. Remember to listen to your body, honor your needs, and seek support when needed as you work toward achieving your health and wellness goals.

CHAPTER 11

DR. BARBARA'S RECIPES FOR MUCUS CLEANSE

1. **Ginger Lemon Detox Drink**:

- **Definition**: A refreshing drink that helps to cleanse the respiratory system and reduce mucus buildup.

- **Ingredients**: Freshly grated ginger, lemon juice, honey, water.

- **How to Prepare**: Boil water, add grated ginger, let it steep for a few minutes, strain, and mix with lemon juice and honey.

- **How to Use**: Consume this drink in the morning on an empty stomach.

- **Dosage**: One cup daily.

- **Side Effects**: Ginger may cause heartburn or stomach upset in some individuals.

- **Precautions**: Avoid if you have gallstones or are on blood-thinning medications.

2. **Turmeric Milk**:

- **Definition**: A warm, soothing beverage that has anti-inflammatory properties and helps clear mucus.

- **Ingredients**: Turmeric powder, milk (or a plant-based alternative), honey.

- **How to Prepare**: Heat milk, stir in turmeric powder and honey until dissolved.

- **How to Use**: Drink before bedtime for maximum benefits.

- **Dosage**: One cup daily.

- **Side Effects**: May cause gastrointestinal upset in some individuals.

- **Precautions**: Avoid if you have gallbladder issues or are on blood-thinning medications.

3. **Apple Cider Vinegar Tonic**:

- **Definition**: A tonic that helps to alkalize the body and reduce mucus production.

- **Ingredients**: Apple cider vinegar, warm water, honey.

- **How to Prepare**: Mix apple cider vinegar with warm water and honey.

- **How to Use**: Drink before meals.

- **Dosage**: One tablespoon of apple cider vinegar diluted in a glass of water, up to three times a day.

- **Side Effects**: May erode tooth enamel and irritate the throat if consumed undiluted.

- **Precautions**: Dilute properly to avoid tooth enamel erosion and throat irritation.

4. **Green Smoothie**:

- **Definition**: A nutrient-rich smoothie that helps to detoxify the body and reduce mucus production.

- **Ingredients**: Spinach, kale, cucumber, green apple, lemon juice, water.

- **How to Prepare**: Blend all ingredients until smooth.

- **How to Use**: Consume as a meal replacement or snack.

- **Dosage**: One serving per day.

- **Side Effects**: None reported.

- **Precautions**: Be cautious if you have thyroid issues, as some greens contain goitrogens which may interfere with thyroid function.

5. **Garlic and Honey Tea**:

- **Definition**: A potent tea that has antimicrobial properties and helps to clear mucus.

- **Ingredients**: Garlic cloves, honey, water.

- **How to Prepare**: Crush garlic cloves, steep in hot water, strain, and add honey.

- **How to Use**: Drink while warm.

- **Dosage**: One cup daily.

- **Side Effects**: May cause heartburn or stomach upset in some individuals.

- **Precautions**: Avoid if you have a bleeding disorder or are on blood-thinning medications.

6. **Vegetable Broth**:

- **Definition**: A nourishing broth that provides essential vitamins and minerals while supporting detoxification.

- **Ingredients**: Various vegetables (carrots, celery, onion, garlic, etc.), water, herbs, spices.

- **How to Prepare**: Simmer vegetables, herbs, and spices in water until flavors are infused, then strain.

- **How to Use**: Drink as a snack or use as a base for soups and stews.

- **Dosage**: As desired.

- **Side Effects**: None reported.

- **Precautions**: None.

7. **Nettle Tea**:

- **Definition**: A herbal tea that acts as a natural antihistamine and helps to reduce mucus production.

- **Ingredients**: Dried nettle leaves, water, honey (optional).

- **How to Prepare**: Steep dried nettle leaves in hot water, strain, and sweeten with honey if desired.

- **How to Use**: Drink 2-3 times a day.

- **Dosage**: One cup, 2-3 times daily.

- **Side Effects**: May cause mild stomach upset or allergic reactions in sensitive individuals.

- **Precautions**: Avoid if pregnant or breastfeeding, or if you have low blood pressure.

8. **Cayenne Pepper Tea**:

- **Definition**: A spicy tea that helps to break up mucus and improve circulation.

- **Ingredients**: Cayenne pepper, lemon juice, water, honey (optional).

- **How to Prepare**: Mix cayenne pepper and lemon juice in hot water, sweeten with honey if desired.

- **How to Use**: Drink while warm.

- **Dosage**: One cup daily.

- **Side Effects**: May cause stomach irritation or allergic reactions in some individuals.

- **Precautions**: Avoid if you have gastrointestinal issues or are sensitive to spicy foods.

9. **Pineapple Cucumber Smoothie**:

- **Definition**: A refreshing smoothie that contains bromelain, an enzyme that helps to reduce mucus.

- **Ingredients**: Pineapple, cucumber, ginger, mint leaves, water.

- **How to Prepare**: Blend all ingredients until smooth.

- **How to Use**: Consume as a snack or meal replacement.

- **Dosage**: One serving per day.

- **Side Effects**: None reported.

- **Precautions**: None.

10. **Peppermint Tea**:

- **Definition**: A soothing tea that helps to clear congestion and alleviate respiratory symptoms.

- **Ingredients**: Peppermint leaves, water, honey (optional).

- **How to Prepare**: Steep peppermint leaves in hot water, strain, and sweeten with honey if desired.

- **How to Use**: Drink 2-3 times a day.

- **Dosage**: One cup, 2-3 times daily.

- **Side Effects**: May cause heartburn or allergic reactions in some individuals.

- **Precautions**: Avoid if you have acid reflux or gastroesophageal reflux disease (GERD).

11. **Lemon Water**:

- **Definition**: A simple and refreshing drink that helps to alkalize the body and reduce mucus production.

- **Ingredients**: Lemon juice, water.

- **How to Prepare**: Mix freshly squeezed lemon juice with water.

- **How to Use**: Drink on an empty stomach in the morning.

- **Dosage**: One glass daily.

- **Side Effects**: May erode tooth enamel if consumed frequently.

- **Precautions**: Rinse mouth with plain water after drinking to protect tooth enamel.

12. **Fennel Seed Tea**:

- **Definition**: A soothing tea that helps to break down mucus and ease respiratory discomfort.

- **Ingredients**: Fennel seeds, water, honey (optional).

- **How to Prepare**: Crush fennel seeds, steep in hot water, strain, and sweeten with honey if desired.

- **How to Use**: Drink 2-3 times a day.

- **Dosage**: One cup, 2-3 times daily.

- **Side Effects**: May cause allergic reactions in some individuals.

- **Precautions**: Avoid if you are allergic to fennel or other plants in the Apiaceae family.

13. **Seaweed Salad**:

- **Definition**: A nutritious salad that contains seaweed, which helps to detoxify the body and reduce mucus production.

- **Ingredients**: Seaweed (such as nori, wakame, or kombu), cucumber, carrot, sesame seeds, rice vinegar, soy sauce, honey.

- **How to Prepare**: Soak seaweed according to package instructions, then toss with sliced vegetables, sesame seeds, rice vinegar, soy sauce, and honey.

- **How to Use**: Serve as a side dish or light meal.

- **Dosage**: As desired.

- **Side Effects**: None reported.

- **Precautions**: Ensure seaweed is sourced from reputable suppliers to avoid contamination with heavy metals or other toxins.

14. **Warm Lemon Water with Cayenne Pepper**:

- **Definition**: A stimulating drink that helps to clear mucus and boost metabolism.

- **Ingredients**: Lemon juice, cayenne pepper, warm water.

- **How to Prepare**: Mix lemon juice and cayenne pepper in warm water.

- **How to Use**: Drink in the morning on an empty stomach.

- **Dosage**: One cup daily.

- **Side Effects**: May cause stomach irritation or heartburn in some individuals.

- **Precautions**: Start with a small amount of cayenne pepper and gradually increase to avoid stomach upset.

15. **Detox Vegetable Soup**:

- **Definition**: A hearty soup packed with detoxifying vegetables and herbs to support mucus clearance.

- **Ingredients**: Various vegetables (carrots, celery, onion, garlic, etc.), vegetable broth, herbs, spices.

- **How to Prepare**: Saute vegetables, then simmer in vegetable broth with herbs and spices until tender.

- **How to Use**: Enjoy as a meal or snack.

- **Dosage**: As desired.

- **Side Effects**: None reported.

- **Precautions**: None.

SOME VITAL HERBAL REMEDIES TO KNOW

Bio Ferro Tonic:

Definition: Bio Ferro Tonic is a dietary supplement primarily composed of herbs and minerals. It's often marketed as a natural way to support overall health, particularly by promoting blood health and circulation.

Ingredients: Typical ingredients in Bio Ferro Tonic may include a blend of herbs such as burdock root, yellow dock root, sarsaparilla root, and cascara sagrada bark, along with minerals like iron and potassium phosphate.

How to Prepare: Bio Ferro Tonic usually comes in liquid form and is typically taken orally. It's important to follow the instructions on the product label for dosage and administration.

Dosage: The dosage can vary depending on the specific product and individual needs. It's crucial to consult with a healthcare professional or follow the recommended dosage on the product label to avoid potential side effects.

How to Use: Bio Ferro Tonic is often taken by adding the recommended dosage to water or juice and consuming it orally. It's important to shake the bottle well before use and store it according to the manufacturer's instructions.

Side Effects: While Bio Ferro Tonic is generally considered safe when used as directed, some individuals may experience side effects such as digestive discomfort, allergic reactions, or interactions with medications. It's essential to consult with a healthcare provider before starting any new supplement regimen, especially if you have underlying health conditions or are taking medications.

Bladderwrack:

Definition: Bladderwrack is a type of seaweed or marine algae commonly used in traditional medicine and as a dietary supplement. It's known for its potential health benefits, particularly related to thyroid health and weight management.

Ingredients: Bladderwrack contains various nutrients, including iodine, vitamins, minerals, and antioxidants. The primary active components are iodine and fucoidan, a type of carbohydrate found in brown seaweeds.

How to Prepare: Bladderwrack supplements are available in various forms, including capsules, powders, and liquid extracts. They can be taken orally with water or added to smoothies and other beverages.

Dosage: The appropriate dosage of bladderwrack can vary based on factors such as age, health status, and the specific product being used. It's essential to follow the recommended dosage on the product label or consult with a healthcare professional for personalized guidance.

How to Use: Bladderwrack supplements are typically taken orally, either with water or mixed into food or beverages. It's important to follow the instructions on the product label and avoid exceeding the recommended dosage.

Side Effects: While bladderwrack is generally considered safe for most people when used in moderation, excessive intake of iodine from bladderwrack supplements can cause thyroid dysfunction and other adverse effects. Individuals with thyroid disorders, iodine sensitivity, or certain medical conditions should exercise caution and consult with a healthcare provider before using bladderwrack supplements. Common side effects may include digestive upset, allergic reactions, or interactions with medications.

Blue Vervain:

Definition: Blue vervain, also known as Verbena hastata, is a perennial herb native to North America. It has been used in traditional medicine for centuries to treat various ailments, including anxiety, insomnia, and digestive issues.

Ingredients: Blue vervain contains several active compounds, including aucubin, verbenalin, and volatile oils. These compounds are believed to contribute to the herb's medicinal properties.

How to Prepare: Blue vervain is typically consumed as a tea or tincture. To make tea, dried blue vervain leaves and flowers are steeped in hot water for several minutes before being strained and consumed. Tinctures are prepared by steeping the herb in alcohol or vinegar to extract its active compounds.

Dosage: The appropriate dosage of blue vervain can vary depending on factors such as age, health status, and the specific preparation being used. It's important to follow the recommended dosage on the product label or consult with a qualified herbalist or healthcare professional for personalized guidance.

How to Use: Blue vervain tea or tincture is typically taken orally. It can be consumed on its own or mixed with honey or other herbal teas for added flavor.

Side Effects: While blue vervain is generally considered safe for most people when used in moderation, excessive intake may cause digestive upset or allergic reactions in some individuals. Pregnant or breastfeeding women should avoid blue vervain due to its potential to stimulate uterine contractions. As with any herbal remedy, it's important to consult with a healthcare provider before using blue vervain, especially if you have underlying health conditions or are taking medications.

Bromide Plus Powder:

Definition: Bromide Plus Powder is a dietary supplement formulated to support thyroid health and promote overall well-being. It typically contains a blend of herbs and minerals that are believed to have beneficial effects on thyroid function.

Ingredients: Bromide Plus Powder often contains a combination of herbs such as bladderwrack, sea moss, and burdock root, along with minerals like iodine and potassium phosphate. These ingredients are thought to support thyroid function and maintain optimal iodine levels in the body.

How to Prepare: Bromide Plus Powder is usually mixed with water or juice to create a drinkable solution. It's important to follow the instructions on the product label for dosage and preparation.

Dosage: The dosage of Bromide Plus Powder can vary depending on the specific product and individual needs. It's crucial to consult with a healthcare professional or follow the recommended dosage on the product label to avoid potential side effects.

How to Use: Bromide Plus Powder is typically taken orally by mixing the recommended dosage with water or juice. It's important to shake or stir the mixture well before consuming it to ensure even distribution of the ingredients.

Side Effects: While Bromide Plus Powder is generally considered safe when used as directed, some individuals may experience side effects such as digestive discomfort or allergic reactions to certain ingredients. It's essential to consult with a healthcare provider before starting any new supplement regimen, especially if you have underlying health conditions or are taking medications.

Bugleweed:

Definition: Bugleweed, also known as Lycopusvirginicus, is a perennial herb native to North America and Europe. It has been used in traditional medicine to treat various conditions, including hyperthyroidism, anxiety, and insomnia.

Ingredients: Bugleweed contains several active compounds, including lithospermic acid, phenolic acids, and flavonoids. These compounds are believed to contribute to the herb's medicinal properties, particularly its ability to regulate thyroid function.

How to Prepare: Bugleweed is commonly consumed as a tea or tincture. To make tea, dried bugleweed leaves and flowers are steeped in hot water for several minutes before being strained and consumed. Tinctures are prepared by steeping the herb in alcohol or vinegar to extract its active compounds.

Dosage: The appropriate dosage of bugleweed can vary depending on factors such as age, health status, and the specific preparation being used. It's important to follow the recommended dosage on the product label or consult with a qualified herbalist or healthcare professional for personalized guidance.

How to Use: Bugleweed tea or tincture is typically taken orally. It can be consumed on its own or mixed with honey or other herbal teas for added flavor.

Side Effects: While bugleweed is generally considered safe for most people when used in moderation, excessive intake may cause digestive upset or allergic reactions in some individuals.

Pregnant or breastfeeding women should avoid bugleweed due to its potential to stimulate uterine contractions. As with any herbal remedy, it's important to consult with a healthcare provider before using bugleweed, especially if you have underlying health conditions or are taking medications.

Burdock:

Definition: Burdock, scientifically known as Arctium lappa, is a biennial plant native to Europe and Asia but now found worldwide. It's part of the Asteraceae family and has been used for centuries in traditional medicine and culinary practices.

Ingredients: Burdock contains various nutrients, including carbohydrates, fiber, vitamins (such as vitamin B6, folate, and vitamin C), and minerals (including potassium, magnesium, and manganese). It also contains active compounds such as polyphenols and volatile oils.

How to Prepare: Burdock can be prepared and consumed in various ways. The roots, leaves, and seeds are all utilized for different purposes. The root is commonly used in cooking, herbal teas, tinctures, and supplements, while the leaves and seeds are sometimes used in herbal preparations.

Dosage: The appropriate dosage of burdock root can vary depending on the specific form and intended use. For culinary purposes, there are no strict dosage guidelines, but for supplements or herbal remedies, it's essential to follow the recommended dosage on the product label or consult with a healthcare professional.

How to Use: Burdock root can be used in cooking by peeling, slicing, and adding it to soups, stews, stir-fries, or salads. It can also be brewed into a tea or used to make tinctures or extracts for medicinal purposes. Some people may also take burdock root supplements in capsule or powder form.

Side Effects: While burdock is generally considered safe for most people when consumed in moderate amounts, some individuals may experience allergic reactions or digestive upset. Additionally, burdock may interact with certain medications or have adverse effects in individuals with certain health conditions, such as diabetes or allergies to plants in the Asteraceae family. It's important to consult with a healthcare provider before using burdock, especially if you have underlying health conditions or are taking medications.

Cascara Sagrada:

Definition: Cascara Sagrada, scientifically known as Rhamnus purshiana, is a species of buckthorn native to western North America. It has been used traditionally as a laxative and to promote bowel regularity.

Ingredients: The primary active ingredients in cascara sagrada are anthraquinone glycosides, particularly cascarosides A and B. These compounds stimulate peristalsis in the colon, leading to increased bowel movements.

How to Prepare: Cascara sagrada is typically prepared as an herbal tea, tincture, or capsule. To make tea, dried cascara sagrada bark is steeped in hot water for several minutes before being strained and consumed. Tinctures are prepared by steeping the bark in alcohol to extract its active compounds.

Dosage: The appropriate dosage of cascara sagrada can vary depending on the specific preparation and intended use. It's important to follow the recommended dosage on the product label or consult with a healthcare professional for personalized guidance.

How to Use: Cascara sagrada tea or tincture is typically taken orally. It's important to start with a low dose and gradually increase if needed to avoid potential side effects such as cramping or diarrhea.

Side Effects: Cascara sagrada is considered safe for short-term use when used as directed. However, long-term or excessive use may lead to dependence, electrolyte imbalance, or dehydration. It may also interact with certain medications or have adverse effects in individuals with certain health conditions. It's important to use cascara sagrada under the guidance of a healthcare professional and to discontinue use if any adverse effects occur.

Cocolmeca:

Definition: Cocolmeca, also known as Smilax ornata or sarsaparilla, is a flowering vine native to Mexico and Central America. It has been used traditionally in Mexican and Central American folk medicine for its purported medicinal properties.

Ingredients: Cocolmeca contains various bioactive compounds, including saponins, flavonoids, and plant sterols. These compounds are believed to contribute to the herb's medicinal properties, including its potential as a diuretic, blood purifier, and anti-inflammatory agent.

How to Prepare: Cocolmeca is commonly prepared and consumed as an herbal tea or decoction. To make tea, dried cocolmeca roots or leaves are steeped in hot water for several minutes before being strained and consumed. Decoctions involve boiling the roots or leaves in water to extract their active compounds.

Dosage: The appropriate dosage of cocolmeca can vary depending on factors such as age, health status, and the specific preparation being used. It's important to follow the recommended dosage on the product label or consult with a qualified herbalist or healthcare professional for personalized guidance.

How to Use: Cocolmeca tea or decoction is typically taken orally. It can also be used topically for certain skin conditions. It's important to use cocolmeca products as directed and to discontinue use if any adverse effects occur.

Side Effects: Cocolmeca is generally considered safe for most people when used in moderate amounts. However, excessive intake may lead to digestive upset or other adverse effects. It may also interact with certain medications or have adverse effects in individuals with certain health conditions. It's important to use cocolmeca under the guidance of a healthcare professional and to discontinue use if any adverse effects occur.

Contribo:

Definition: Contribo, also known as Aristolochiatrilobata, is a vine native to the Caribbean and Central America. It has been used traditionally in folk medicine for various purposes, including as a remedy for digestive issues, inflammation, and pain relief.

Ingredients: Contribo contains several bioactive compounds, including aristolochic acids, flavonoids, and alkaloids. These compounds are believed to contribute to the herb's medicinal properties, including its potential as an anti-inflammatory and analgesic agent.

How to Prepare: Contribo is typically prepared and consumed as an herbal tea or decoction. To make tea, dried contribo leaves or stems are steeped in hot water for several minutes before being strained and consumed. Decoctions involve boiling the leaves or stems in water to extract their active compounds.

Dosage: The appropriate dosage of contribo can vary depending on factors such as age, health status, and the specific preparation being used. It's important to follow the recommended dosage on the product label or consult with a qualified herbalist or healthcare professional for personalized guidance.

How to Use: Contribo tea or decoction is typically taken orally. It's important to use contribo products as directed and to discontinue use if any adverse effects occur.

Side Effects: Contribo contains aristolochic acids, which have been associated with serious adverse effects, including kidney damage and cancer. Due to these safety concerns, the use of contribo is highly discouraged, and it's important to avoid products containing aristolochic acids. Individuals should seek alternative remedies for their health needs.

Dandelion Root:

Definition: Dandelion, scientifically known as Taraxacum officinale, is a common flowering plant found worldwide. While often considered a pesky weed, dandelion has a long history of use in traditional medicine for its various health benefits.

Ingredients: Dandelion root contains several bioactive compounds, including sesquiterpene lactones, triterpenes, flavonoids, and polysaccharides. These compounds are believed to contribute to the herb's medicinal properties, including its potential as a diuretic, digestive aid, and liver tonic.

How to Prepare: Dandelion root can be prepared and consumed in various forms, including teas, tinctures, capsules, and extracts. To make tea, dried dandelion root is steeped in hot water for several minutes before being strained and consumed. Tinctures are prepared by steeping the root in alcohol or vinegar to extract its active compounds.

Dosage: The appropriate dosage of dandelion root can vary depending on factors such as age, health status, and the specific preparation being used. It's important to follow the recommended dosage on the product label or consult with a qualified herbalist or healthcare professional for personalized guidance.

How to Use: Dandelion root tea, tincture, or capsules are typically taken orally. It's important to use dandelion root products as directed and to discontinue use if any adverse effects occur.

Side Effects: Dandelion root is generally considered safe for most people when used in moderate amounts. However, some individuals may experience allergic reactions or digestive upset. It may also interact with certain medications or have adverse effects in individuals with certain health conditions. It's important to use dandelion root under the guidance of a healthcare professional and to discontinue use if any adverse effects occur.

Green Food Plus:

Definition: Green Food Plus is a dietary supplement formulated to provide a concentrated source of nutrients derived from various green plants. It's designed to support overall health and well-being by delivering essential vitamins, minerals, antioxidants, and phytonutrients.

Ingredients: Green Food Plus typically contains a blend of powdered green vegetables, grasses, algae, and other plant-based ingredients. Common ingredients may include wheatgrass, barley grass, spirulina, chlorella, alfalfa, kale, spinach, and broccoli, among others.

How to Prepare: Green Food Plus is usually available in powder form and can be mixed with water, juice, or smoothies. It's important to follow the recommended dosage on the product label and to consume it as part of a balanced diet.

Dosage: The appropriate dosage of Green Food Plus can vary depending on the specific product and individual needs. It's important to follow the recommended dosage on the product label or consult with a healthcare professional for personalized guidance.

How to Use: Green Food Plus powder is typically mixed with water, juice, or smoothies and consumed orally. It's often taken once or twice daily, preferably with meals, to maximize nutrient absorption.

Side Effects: Green Food Plus is generally considered safe for most people when used as directed. However, some individuals may experience digestive upset or allergic reactions to certain ingredients. It's important to consult with a healthcare provider before starting any new supplement regimen, especially if you have underlying health conditions or are taking medications.

Guaco:

Definition: Guaco, also known as Mikania cordata or Mikania glomerata, is a medicinal plant native to Central and South America. It has a long history of use in traditional medicine for its potential therapeutic properties.

Ingredients: Guaco contains several bioactive compounds, including coumarins, flavonoids, tannins, and saponins. These compounds are believed to contribute to the herb's medicinal properties, including its potential as an expectorant, anti-inflammatory, and antispasmodic agent.

How to Prepare: Guaco is typically prepared and consumed as an herbal tea or infusion. To make tea, dried guaco leaves are steeped in hot water for several minutes before being strained and consumed.

Dosage: The appropriate dosage of guaco can vary depending on factors such as age, health status, and the specific preparation being used. It's important to follow the recommended dosage on the product label or consult with a qualified herbalist or healthcare professional for personalized guidance.

How to Use: Guaco tea is typically taken orally. It can be consumed on its own or mixed with honey or other herbal teas for added flavor.

Side Effects: Guaco is generally considered safe for most people when used in moderate amounts. However, some individuals may experience allergic reactions or digestive upset. It may also interact with certain medications or have adverse effects in individuals with certain health conditions. It's important to use guaco under the guidance of a healthcare professional and to discontinue use if any adverse effects occur.

Irish Sea Moss:

Definition: Irish Sea Moss is a term often used interchangeably with Irish Moss, referring to the same species of red algae, Chondrus crispus. It's harvested from the rocky shores of the Atlantic coastlines of Europe and North America.

Ingredients: Irish Sea Moss shares the same nutritional profile as Irish Moss, containing iodine, vitamins, minerals, and polysaccharides. It's valued for its potential health benefits, including supporting thyroid function, boosting immune health, and promoting digestion.

How to Prepare: Irish Sea Moss is prepared in the same way as Irish Moss, by soaking it in water to rehydrate and soften it before use. It can be used in culinary applications or consumed as a dietary supplement.

Dosage: The dosage of Irish Sea Moss depends on the form and intended use. As a dietary supplement, it's important to follow the recommended dosage on the product label or consult with a healthcare professional for personalized guidance.

How to Use: Irish Sea Moss can be used in various culinary applications, including soups, smoothies, desserts, and sauces. It can also be consumed as a dietary supplement in the form of capsules, powders, or extracts.

Side Effects: Similar to Irish Moss, Irish Sea Moss is generally considered safe for most people when consumed in moderate amounts. However, individuals with seaweed allergies or sensitivities to carrageenan should exercise caution. It's important to discontinue use if any adverse effects occur and to consult with a healthcare professional if you have any concerns.

Lymphalin:

Definition: Lymphalin is a herbal supplement formulated to support lymphatic system health. The lymphatic system plays a crucial role in immune function and waste removal in the body, and Lymphalin is designed to promote its proper function.

Ingredients: Lymphalin typically contains a blend of herbs and botanical extracts known for their traditional use in supporting lymphatic system health. Common ingredients may include cleavers, red clover, echinacea, burdock root, and calendula, among others.

How to Prepare: Lymphalin is usually available in capsule or liquid form. Capsules are taken orally with water, while liquid forms may be mixed with water or juice before consumption. It's important to follow the recommended dosage on the product label.

Dosage: The appropriate dosage of Lymphalin can vary depending on the specific product and individual needs. It's important to follow the recommended dosage on the product label or consult with a healthcare professional for personalized guidance.

How to Use: Lymphalin capsules are typically taken orally with water, while liquid forms may be mixed with water or juice before consumption. It's often recommended to take Lymphalin on an empty stomach for optimal absorption.

Side Effects: Lymphalin is generally considered safe for most people when used as directed. However, some individuals may experience mild side effects such as gastrointestinal discomfort or allergic reactions to certain ingredients. It's important to consult with a healthcare provider before starting any new supplement regimen, especially if you have underlying health conditions or are taking medications.

Manjakani:

Definition: Manjakani, also known as Quercus infectoria or oak gall, is a natural substance derived from the oak tree. It has been used for centuries in traditional medicine for its potential health benefits, particularly for women's health and vaginal tightening.

Ingredients: Manjakani contains various bioactive compounds, including tannins, flavonoids, and gallic acid. These compounds are believed to contribute to the herb's medicinal properties, including its potential as an astringent and antiseptic agent.

How to Prepare: Manjakani is typically available in powder, capsule, or liquid extract form. It can be taken orally or used topically depending on the intended use. For vaginal tightening, manjakani may be applied topically as a gel or inserted into the vagina in capsule form.

Dosage: The appropriate dosage of manjakani can vary depending on factors such as age, health status, and the specific preparation being used. It's important to follow the recommended dosage on the product label or consult with a qualified herbalist or healthcare professional for personalized guidance.

How to Use: Manjakani can be taken orally or used topically depending on the intended use. It's important to use manjakani products as directed and to discontinue use if any adverse effects occur.

Side Effects: Manjakani is generally considered safe for most people when used in moderate amounts. However, some individuals may experience allergic reactions or skin irritation when used topically. It's important to use manjakani under the guidance of a healthcare professional and to discontinue use if any adverse effects occur.

Red Clover:

Definition: Red clover, scientifically known as Trifolium pratense, is a flowering plant belonging to the legume family. It's native to Europe, Western Asia, and Northwest Africa but has been naturalized in many other regions. Red clover has been used in traditional medicine for various purposes, including its potential to support women's health and menopausal symptoms.

Ingredients: Red clover contains several bioactive compounds, including isoflavones (such as genistein and daidzein), flavonoids, and phytoestrogens. These compounds are believed to contribute to the herb's medicinal properties, including its potential as a hormone-balancing agent and its ability to support cardiovascular health.

How to Prepare: Red clover is typically prepared and consumed as an herbal tea or tincture. To make tea, dried red clover flowers are steeped in hot water for several minutes before being strained and consumed. Tinctures are prepared by steeping the flowers in alcohol or vinegar to extract their active compounds.

Dosage: The appropriate dosage of red clover can vary depending on factors such as age, health status, and the specific preparation being used. It's important to follow the recommended dosage on the product label or consult with a qualified herbalist or healthcare professional for personalized guidance.

How to Use: Red clover tea or tincture is typically taken orally. It's important to use red clover products as directed and to discontinue use if any adverse effects occur.

Side Effects: Red clover is generally considered safe for most people when used in moderate amounts. However, some individuals may experience allergic reactions or digestive upset. It may also interact with certain medications or have adverse effects in individuals with certain health conditions. It's important to use red clover under the guidance of a healthcare professional and to discontinue use if any adverse effects occur.

Herban Iron:

Definition: Herban Iron is a dietary supplement designed to provide an easily absorbable form of iron to support healthy iron levels in the body. It's particularly beneficial for individuals with iron deficiency or anemia.

Ingredients: Herban Iron typically contains iron in the form of ferrous bisglycinate, which is a highly bioavailable and gentle form of iron that is less likely to cause digestive upset or constipation compared to other forms of iron. It may also contain other ingredients such as vitamin C to enhance iron absorption.

How to Prepare: Herban Iron is usually available in capsule or liquid form. Capsules are taken orally with water, while liquid forms may be mixed with water or juice before consumption. It's important to follow the recommended dosage on the product label.

Dosage: The appropriate dosage of Herban Iron depends on factors such as age, gender, and the severity of iron deficiency. It's important to consult with a healthcare professional to determine the correct dosage for individual needs.

How to Use: Herban Iron capsules are typically taken orally with water, while liquid forms may be mixed with water or juice before consumption. It's important to take Herban Iron as directed and to avoid taking it with dairy products, antacids, or other substances that may interfere with iron absorption.

Side Effects: While Herban Iron is generally considered safe for most people when used as directed, some individuals may experience mild side effects such as gastrointestinal discomfort or constipation. It's important to consult with a healthcare professional before starting any new supplement regimen, especially if you have underlying health conditions or are taking medications.

Hydrangea:

Definition: Hydrangea, scientifically known as Hydrangea arborescens, is a flowering shrub native to North America. It has been used traditionally in herbal medicine for its potential diuretic and anti-inflammatory properties.

Ingredients: Hydrangea contains several bioactive compounds, including saponins, flavonoids, and glycosides. These compounds are believed to contribute to the herb's medicinal properties, including its potential as a diuretic, kidney tonic, and anti-inflammatory agent.

How to Prepare: Hydrangea root is typically prepared and consumed as an herbal tea or tincture. To make tea, dried hydrangea root is steeped in hot water for several minutes before being strained and consumed. Tinctures are prepared by steeping the root in alcohol or vinegar to extract its active compounds.

Dosage: The appropriate dosage of hydrangea can vary depending on factors such as age, health status, and the specific preparation being used. It's important to follow the recommended dosage on the product label or consult with a qualified herbalist or healthcare professional for personalized guidance.

How to Use: Hydrangea tea or tincture is typically taken orally. It's important to use hydrangea products as directed and to discontinue use if any adverse effects occur.

Side Effects: Hydrangea is generally considered safe for most people when used in moderate amounts. However, some individuals may experience digestive upset or allergic reactions. It may also interact with certain medications or have adverse effects in individuals with certain health conditions. It's important to use hydrangea under the guidance of a healthcare professional and to discontinue use if any adverse effects occur.

Irish Moss:

Definition: Irish Moss, scientifically known as Chondrus crispus, is a species of red algae or seaweed native to the Atlantic coastlines of Europe and North America. It has been used for centuries in traditional Irish and Scottish cuisine, as well as in herbal medicine.

Ingredients: Irish Moss is rich in various nutrients, including iodine, sulfur compounds, vitamins (such as vitamin A, vitamin K, and vitamin B12), minerals (including calcium, magnesium, potassium, and sodium), and polysaccharides (such as carrageenan). These nutrients are believed to contribute to the herb's potential health benefits.

How to Prepare: Irish Moss is typically prepared by soaking it in water to rehydrate and soften it before use. It can be added to soups, stews, smoothies, desserts, and other dishes as a thickening agent or nutritional supplement.

Dosage: The appropriate dosage of Irish Moss can vary depending on factors such as age, health status, and the specific preparation being used. It's important to follow recipes or guidelines for culinary use and to consult with a healthcare professional for guidance on using Irish Moss as a dietary supplement.

How to Use: Irish Moss can be used in culinary applications to add thickness and nutritional value to dishes. It can also be consumed as a dietary supplement in the form of capsules, powders, or extracts.

Side Effects: Irish Moss is generally considered safe for most people when consumed in moderate amounts as part of a balanced diet. However, some individuals may be allergic to seaweed or carrageenan, a compound found in Irish Moss that is used as a food additive. It's important to discontinue use if any adverse effects occur and to consult with a healthcare professional if you have any concerns.

Cell Food:

Definition: Cell Food is a dietary supplement marketed as a highly oxygenating and alkalizing formula. It's claimed to support overall health and vitality by providing essential nutrients and oxygen to the cells.

Ingredients: The exact ingredients of Cell Food can vary depending on the brand, but it typically contains a proprietary blend of minerals, enzymes, electrolytes, and trace elements. Some common ingredients may include purified water, dissolved oxygen, seawater extract, and plant-based enzymes.

How to Prepare: Cell Food is usually available in liquid form and is typically taken orally. It can be consumed directly or diluted in water or juice before consumption.

Dosage: The dosage of Cell Food can vary depending on the specific product and individual needs. It's important to follow the recommended dosage on the product label or consult with a healthcare professional for personalized guidance.

How to Use: Cell Food is typically taken orally, either directly or mixed into water or juice. It's important to shake the bottle well before use and to store it according to the manufacturer's instructions.

Side Effects: Cell Food is generally considered safe for most people when used as directed. However, some individuals may experience mild digestive upset or allergic reactions to certain ingredients. It's essential to consult with a healthcare provider before starting any new supplement regimen, especially if you have underlying health conditions or are taking medications.

Chaparral:

Definition: Chaparral, scientifically known as Larrea tridentata, is a shrub native to the southwestern United States and northern Mexico. It has been used for centuries by Native American tribes for its medicinal properties and is commonly used in herbal medicine today.

Ingredients: Chaparral contains several bioactive compounds, including nordihydroguaiaretic acid (NDGA), flavonoids, lignans, and volatile oils. NDGA is believed to be the primary active compound responsible for many of chaparral's therapeutic effects.

How to Prepare: Chaparral can be prepared and consumed in various forms, including teas, tinctures, capsules, and topical preparations. To make tea, dried chaparral leaves are steeped in hot water for several minutes before being strained and consumed. Tinctures are prepared by steeping the herb in alcohol or vinegar to extract its active compounds.

Dosage: The appropriate dosage of chaparral can vary depending on the specific form and intended use. It's important to follow the recommended dosage on the product label or consult with a healthcare professional for personalized guidance.

How to Use: Chaparral tea or tincture is typically taken orally. It can also be applied topically to the skin for certain conditions. It's important to use chaparral products as directed and to discontinue use if any adverse effects occur.

Side Effects: Chaparral is generally considered safe for most people when used in moderate amounts. However, excessive intake or prolonged use may lead to liver toxicity or other adverse effects. It may also interact with certain medications or have adverse effects in individuals with certain health conditions. It's important to use chaparral under the guidance of a healthcare professional and to discontinue use if any adverse effects occur.

Blood Purifier:

Definition: Blood purifiers are herbal remedies or dietary supplements believed to cleanse or detoxify the blood, often promoting overall health and well-being. They are thought to support the body's natural detoxification processes and improve blood circulation.

Ingredients: Blood purifiers may contain a variety of herbs and botanical extracts known for their purported cleansing and detoxifying properties. Common ingredients include burdock root, red clover, dandelion root, and yellow dock root, among others.

How to Prepare: Blood purifiers are typically available in various forms, including capsules, tablets, powders, and liquid extracts. They are usually taken orally with water or juice, following the recommended dosage on the product label.

Dosage: The dosage of blood purifiers can vary depending on the specific product and individual needs. It's important to adhere to the recommended dosage on the product label or consult with a healthcare professional for personalized guidance.

How to Use: Blood purifiers are typically taken orally, either with water or mixed into beverages. They are often used as part of a detoxification regimen or to support overall health and vitality.

Side Effects: While blood purifiers are generally considered safe for most people when used as directed, some individuals may experience side effects such as digestive discomfort, allergic reactions, or interactions with medications. It's important to consult with a healthcare provider before starting any new supplement regimen, especially if you have underlying health conditions or are taking medications.

THE END